DEDICATION

This book is dedicated to all ladies who want to look their best.
This book is for you. You are beautiful.

TABLE OF CONTENTS

Beauty Essentials for Her

How to Look Fab and Glam in an Instant

By: Sharon Douglas

9781635010060

PUBLISHERS NOTES

Disclaimer – Speedy Publishing LLC

This publication is intended to provide helpful and informative material. It is not intended to diagnose, treat, cure, or prevent any health problem or condition, nor is intended to replace the advice of a physician. No action should be taken solely on the contents of this book. Always consult your physician or qualified health-care professional on any matters regarding your health and before adopting any suggestions in this book or drawing inferences from it.

The author and publisher specifically disclaim all responsibility for any liability, loss or risk, personal or otherwise, which is incurred as a consequence, directly or indirectly, from the use or application of any contents of this book.

Any and all product names referenced within this book are the trademarks of their respective owners. None of these owners have sponsored, authorized, endorsed, or approved this book.

Always read all information provided by the manufacturers' product labels before using their products. The author and publisher are not responsible for claims made by manufacturers.

This book was originally printed before 2014. This is an adapted reprint by Speedy Publishing LLC with newly updated content designed to help readers with much more accurate and timely information and data.

Speedy Publishing LLC

40 E Main Street, Newark, Delaware, 19711

Contact Us: 1-888-248-4521

Website: http://www.speedypublishing.co

REPRINTED Paperback Edition: ISBN: 9781635010060

Manufactured in the United States of America

Chapter 1- The Basic Beauty Essentials

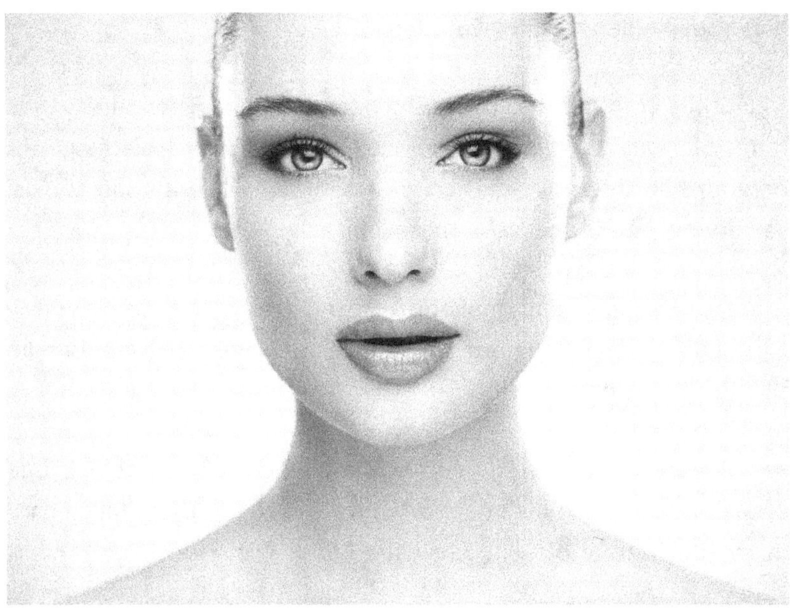

Individuals who have great looking hands are more likely to have hands that people want to hold. Perhaps your wedding is coming up. There is no telling the number of people who will want to see your ring and in turn get to see your hands. On the other hand, you may find that your hands are the focus of pictures. You will need to take steps to ensure that your hands look great. Even if it is not your wedding, you want to take a bit of time to take care of your hands.

What About Them?

You may be wondering, what elements of your hands should you be concerned with? When it comes to beauty tips, people often do not think about their hands, but if you have ever shaken the hand of someone who has bad skin or otherwise poor hands, you likely have remembered it. Here are some tips to help you to improve the quality of the skin on your hands.

• Wash hands properly and often. When it comes to keeping your hands healthy, one of the first steps is t keep them clean. Use a nail brush under your nails and on top of them. Use a quality, but not harsh soap when washing your hands.

• Limit the amount of alcohol used on your hands. There are a wide range of products that, with one squirt, are able to kill all the germs on your hands. Many are alcohol based and while a good choice, can dry out your hands. Use these limitedly.

• Do use lotions and moisturizer. The hands are continuously exposed and need a layer of moisturizer to protect the hands from the harsh elements it meets.

• Tackle skin problems. If you have any type of skin problem, one of the best things you can do for yourself is to get them taken care of by your dermatologist. Since the hands are so exposed, this is very important.

When it comes to your hands, do take care of them. This will make a considerable difference in the quality of your skin overall too and it can prevent you from illnesses since nail beds are one of the worst places for bacteria and pathogens to lurk. Take time to consider your hands: they do matter in terms of what your first impression is with individuals you are just meeting.

7 Things To Do For Natural Beauty

Natural beauty is the best type of beauty. It is recognized by many to be the most amazing and pleasing form. Plus, when you are beautiful, you have a better self image and you have a better outlook on life. The key is being able to do this. For those who want to have a natural beauty, it is always best to make wise decisions about their beauty region. The following are some of the most important things to do when looking for beautiful, natural skin and overall beauty.

1. Care for you face with love: use only those products for your face and skin that are all natural. Organic products are even better. Doing this will aid you in having amazing looking skin for the long term.

2. Keep your skin hydrated. To do this, you will need to consume a least eight full glasses of water each day. You may want to drink juices too as they often have natural nutrients in them. Yet, water is the key to health.

3. Make sure each meal has a wide range of colorful vegetables and fruits in it. You need the antioxidants to improve the quality of skin and to flush out the debris and plague from your arteries and skin cells.

4. Choose concealers based on the ingredient they have in them. You will want to choose products that provide the most natural base since these items are so close to the skin.

5. Always use UV protection make up. Or apply a layer of UV sunscreen under your make up and regularly apply again throughout the course of the day. Even in the winter time, you need to protect your skin from the harm that the sun can cause. Up to 80 percent of skin damage comes from the sun.

6. Apply less make up overall to cover your face. You will want to keep your make up fresh ad light in color. Use naturally based colors for the best overall results.

7. Keep your eye on trends, but go with what you love. Make up color trends change often. New products hit the market each season. Your job is to choose those that give you the best look.

When you incorporate these tips into your overall beauty regimen, you will see marked improvement in your overall skin quality and your look. Keep it up and you will be fighting aging too.

A Healthy Diet Leads To Healthy Skin

What does your diet do for your skin's health? If you are eating a well balanced diet, you may be impressed with the quality of your skin. The two interact with each other, just like every other organ in your body performs only as well as the nutrients it is provided. When it comes to eating healthy, there are several things to keep in mind in terms of what you should eat to help improve your skin quality. In fact, your skin is a direct reflection of the quality of foods you do consume.

Hydration Is Number One

Before looking any further, remember this. In order for your body to have healthy skin, each of the skin cells needs to provide with enough water. There is no easier way to do this than to just drink enough water each day. What you may not realize, too, is that water plays an extra role in the process of keeping skin looking young. It aid in flushing away all of the cells that have died. This helps to keep your outside layer of skin as healthy as it can possibly be.

Antioxidants Are Essential

If you are hoping for a way to help reduce the signs of aging, you can do so through antioxidants. Antioxidants are the very powerful elements that are found in vegetables. They work to keep skin cells as healthy as possible. These are the cleaners of the body. They work to remove waste product from cells which in turn allows the skin to remain great looking. Antioxidants are a type of exfoliation for the skin that comes from the inside out. They also are great at removing build up in your arteries and blood vessels, which can prevent cancers and aid in the removal of dead cells.

To get these benefits, eat a diet that is rich in antioxidants. Choose vegetables and fruits that have deep colors. For example, deep greens are important. Choose a wide range of colors, too. Yellow squashes, orange melons, and blueberries are full of antioxidants that can provide this benefit to your skin.

When it comes to your diet, it does play a role in the health of your skin. There is never a time when you want to consider over the counter medications and anti aging products if you have not taken the time to improve the quality of your diet. Your diet has a direct affect on the quality of your skin.

Caring For Hair: All Those Products

Most individuals spend a decent amount of money on hair care products each month. If you are spending a great deal on these products, you may be shocked to learn that you can get many of the same quality products for less. Plus, you also have to take into consideration what you actually need to use. Finally, keep in mind that using too many products can really damage your hair. So, what is the solution to all of these problems and still allows you to have great hair?

One option to consider is simply purchasing only what you need and working towards having healthier hair. For example, you may think you need mousse, gels and other hair styling products, but in fact healthy hair may not require nearly as much product. A good example of this is products that add nothing but shine to the hair. You can add them to your hair, or instead, you can simply ensure that your hair is well cared. Do not over wash and get great resets that way.

In addition to this consideration, keep in mind what you are actually putting on your hair. Adding toxic chemicals and sprays to your hair is made worse when you spend hours a month blow drying it. The best result here is to simply reduce the amount of chemicals added. You may even want to consider finding a few organic products. These work well and do not hurt your hair in the process.

Here are a few more tips to keep in mind:

• Don't wash your hair every day. You do not need to and it strips many of the nutrients from your hair you need.

• Use minimal amounts of any product that you do use. Follow the directions on the product. Chances are good that you need far less than you are using.

• Switch out conditioners and shampoos every few months. These are often leaving their own residue in your hair and after a while it can build up. Switching to another brand product every few months will help you get a great clean feeling.

Minimize the use of your hair dryer, too. This too aids in the breakdown of your hair. Most importantly, take care of it. Don't keep it up in a pony tail and be sure that you are spending some time having it professionally cut. All of these small things add up to very impressive hair.

Beginner Beauty Tips

It does not matter if you are 40 and hoping to get back into the habit of wearing makeup or if you are 13 and just starting out. The key is to have great looking skin and features. To help you to do so, keep in mind a few of the most important beauty secrets when it comes to all aspects of beautification of your body. Each person is different and your tastes are important too. Keep in mind that you want to be proud of the way you look.

#1: Choose Quality Products

You do not have to purchase the most expensive beauty products on the market and you most definitely do not need to invest in over priced items that will help your face look younger. Instead, choose quality, middle of the road products that are within your budget. If you are unsure what type of products to buy, have a professional aid you. Have them help you to choose the best make up products for your face.

#2: Less Is More

When it comes to make up, today's biggest trend is less is more. You still need make up but you just might need less. People expect you to look natural and the skin will only look as good as the makeup you apply to it. Keep your make up less caking and more powder and soft. You want to create a natural beauty, not a makeup beauty.

#3: Take Care of It All

Your make up, your nail polish and your pedicures all matter. In order to have that complete look where you stand out as the next beauty queen, you really do need to pay attention to all aspects of your body. If you plan to wear sandals or other open toe shoes, get a pedicure. If you have not had a manicure in the last dozen years, now is the right time. Go and have your eye brows professionally done. Doing all of these things may seem like a lot of work, but really, it just adds to the overall quality of your look.

When you take the time to apply these tips, your beauty will skyrocket. Individuals will be impressed with the quality of your look and overall, you could find yourself more confident and happy about your overall look too. Don't overdo it. Moreover, most importantly, seek out help if you need it.

Caring For Your Nails

If you are like most people, you spend your days working with your hands. You clean with them; you cook with them you spend hours pounding away at a keyboard using them. The problem happens when your nails begin to show damage for all that you do to them. If you are hoping to have great looking nails for a long time, you will need to invest some serious attention in your nail care. The good news is that it does not have to be a hard process to follow.

Start with a good cleaning. Use a nail brush for the hard to reach underside of your nails. You also want to focus on the tops of the nails, giving them a once over with the brush to loosen and remove any debris or dead skin cells there. Next, use a cuticle trimmer to push back and trim those cuticles. This aids you in having great looking nails but it also helps the nails to grow back faster and better. You will want to be careful not to cut yourself here as that is worse than having the cuticles in the first place. Also, remove any hangnails you have.

Do invest in manicures and pedicures. Pedicures do clean up your nails as mentioned above, but they also help to moisturize the nails and add good nutrients to the nails and the surround tissue. This is beneficial to your overall look. Also, consider having a professional pedicure and manicure at least one time every month. This makes an incredible difference in your nail care.

When choosing products to apply to your nails, you should keep these things in mind.

• Choose a product that is as healthy as possible. Some nail polishes and other applications are available as organic or less toxic versions. It does make a difference!

• Choose products that are middle of the line in terms of costs. Quality is important for a professional look.

• Choose colors and styles that you like. After all, you do want to enjoy those nails yourself.

Keeping up with your nails does not have to be difficult. Invest just a few minutes each day for touch ups and about an hour once a week and you will have some of the most amazing looking nails in your area. Moreover, you can definitely count on quality if you do take care of your nails on a regular basis.

Choosing The Right Nail Salon

There are many nail salons located in most larger cities. Even smaller cities have a few. Many of these salons are a great choice, the ideal location to have your manicure and pedicure done. If you are in the search for a new location to get your nails done, it may pay off to take some time to consider all of your options. Finding the right salon means taking into consideration cost and the number of services offered. It also means paying attention to the cleanliness and the friendliness of the staff. After all, there is likely another salon to choose from if this one does not fit your bill.

First: Cleanliness

One of the most important first steps in the process of selecting a nail salon is finding an establishment that is clean and well kept. The amount of bacteria and other pathogens found on finger and toe nails is considerable. Therefore, you do need to take into consideration how well the place is maintained. Many states and counties do require that nail facilities are inspected once or twice a year, most of the time these unannounced visits. Contact your local health board to find out if this is done and if so, what the results where for your favorite locations. In many cases, it will be eye opening.

Comparing Service and Costs

The next important features when it comes to finding the right nail salon are friendliness and the cost of the services. Here are a few tips to keep in mind.

1. Choose a nail salon that offers or specializes in the services you are hoping for. Air brushing, for example, is a skill that is learned. You will not get the same results from all salons.

2. Next, consider how they handle you when you are getting your nails done. Are they rough? Do you enjoy speaking with them? If not, consider an alternative location.

3. Be sure you are comfortable within the prices they have. If the salon is established and highly expensive, consider a nail salon that is less costly. You may find that they are just as capable but have lower prices.

Not all nail salons are the same. Do take the time to find the one that is able to meet all of your needs. The good news is that once you find the right salon, chances are good that your nails will look fabulous and you will love going there.

Contact Lenses and Beauty

Are you tired of wearing glasses but feel as though you can't get into contacts? Or, perhaps you are hoping to change the color of your eyes. Contact lenses have come a long way in recent years. These products are very versatile and they are healthy for your eyes, healthier than any of the older products were.

Plus, more people than ever are able to use contact lenses. Even those that were once told that they could not, are now able to fit nicely into a pair of contact lenses. Of course, there is nothing wrong with wearing glasses, but if you want to highlight your eyes with makeup and you want to look a bit trendier, find out if you can use contact lenses to help you accomplish this.

Contact lenses were designed to aid in improving the eye sight of individuals who did not want to or could not wear glasses. The earlier products were hard, literally, and they often were uncomfortable in the eye. The contact lenses of today are soft, flexible lenses that are easily fit into the eye and easy to maintain.

You will also find that they don't feel like anything. In fact, it is unlikely that you will actually feel the lens in your eye after the first few minutes. The numbers of different styles are available to aid in making the contacts feel comfortable. There are products that are likely to keep your eyes very moist and comfortable.

Now, it is even possible to wear contact lenses just to change the eye color. In fact, you can even choose from a wide range of different products that can mask what your eyes look like. For natural beauty, though, you will want to consider eye colors that are suitable for you and that you can pull off.

For example, if you have very dark brown eyes, you likely will only be able to apply a contact lens that can slightly change the color of your eye. On the other hand, those who have eyes that are light blue will be able to change their eye color to virtually anything.

The only stipulation of using contact lenses either to stop wearing glasses or for cosmetic reasons is that you need to keep them clean. They can be slightly labor intensive, but the underlying benefit is that they can change your entire look with just a few seconds.

CHAPTER 2- BEAUTY AND THE FIRST IMPRESSION

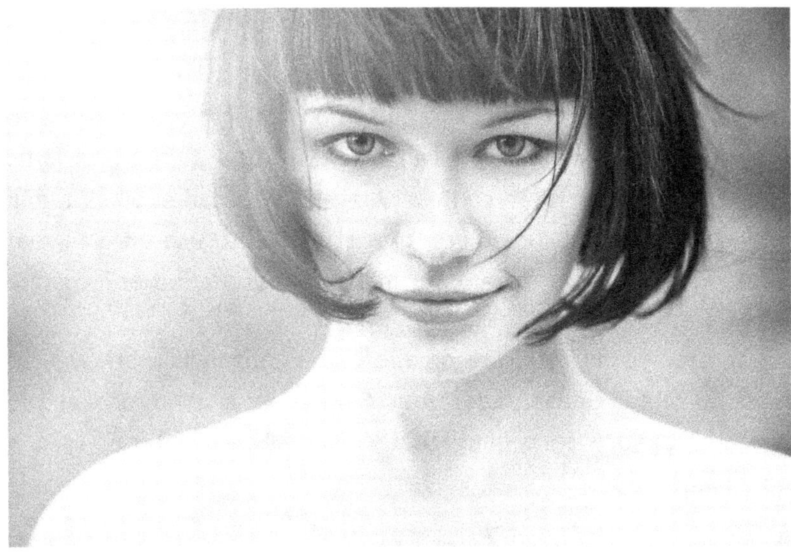

The dreaded look in the mirror shows the dark circles under your eyes. What are you supposed to do about it? If you have to look great, there may be a few ways that you can greatly improve these dark circles under your eyes.

What causes them to happen? Sometimes this is hereditary, and there is very little you can do about those dark circles. They can also be caused by a lack of sleep or not getting enough water. Dehydration is one of the key and most common reasons for dark circles under the eyes.

Naturally Get Rid Of Them

Of course, the most important way to get rid of dark circles is to get more sleep and to drink more water. This process can take some time, though.

You'll need a few hours of sleep and you should try to drink up to eight glasses of water each day. Look for all natural skin care products, too.

These can give you a lot of help in hiding the dark circles when you are unable to otherwise improve them. A good place to start is with a natural moisturizer. This aids in providing more moisture to the skin in this area which can cause the dark circles to fade. Look for products that contain Vitamin K, sesame oil, Vitamin E and avocado oil. These are a great choice to use on a regular basis, too, especially under your make up if you are prone to dark circles.

A variety of concealers are on the market that will work well to mask the dark circles under your eyes. Take a good look at the product. Choose something that is actually all natural, if it is possible to do so.

Do make sure to choose the right color concealer. If you do not, you could risk making the dark circles stand out more so. Choose a natural color that matches your skin well. Or, choose a concealer that is just one shade lighter than your foundation. This will give you the best results in hiding the dark circles under your eyes.

When it comes to hiding your dark circles, keep in mind that there are many ways to do so, but the best way is to take steps to help you to stop them from happening. In other words, get some sleep and drink water, too. Your beautiful skin does not need to be marred by dark circles.

Chapped Lips? How To Avoid This Problem

Chapped lips are one of the first signs of the winter months and they can be one of the most difficult health problems to overcome. When your lips are chapped, you want to wet them over and over again since this action actually seems to sooth them. The problem is, as they dry, the wetting them has made them worse. What can you do to overcome this? In addition, what options are there for avoiding dry lips in the first place?

Treating Chapped Lips

As a fashion statement or a beauty statement, there is o doubt that chapped lips are a big no-no. The pealing and the pain they cause are going to make any lipstick that you apply over them hard to remove and horrible to look at.

You may even get a burning sensation if you tried to cover them up. The best way to treat them is with a soothing, medicated chap stick or lip balm. These are found at most location where medications are sold. Avoid products that are sugar based or that are made for children. What you are looking for is a specific, medicated product that will place a very small dose of medication into these wounds to help them heal. They also work to lock in the moisture on your lips. Apply as often as needed until the painful cracks have healed.

Avoiding It

The only thing better than improving chapped lips is to actually be able to avoid getting them. In many cases, you can do this. First, be sure you stay hydrated. If your body is not hydrated the skin, and the lip, cells will become dry, leaving them highly vulnerable to wind and cold weather.

Second, cover up. When heading outdoors in the cold weather, wear a scarf around your face. This is especially true of very low temperatures, also when the wind is blowing.

Next, apply a layer of moisture protection to your lips. Choose a lip balm, not necessarily one that is medicated, to keep your lips moist. These products are important because of the close proximity to your mouth (the moisture there is what ends up causing the chapped feeling.)

Stop licking your lips. Avoid having this big beauty problem. Simply treat your lips with these products so that you can use lipsticks again. You should avoid these products if you have chapped lips since they can worsen the situation.

Foods For Great Looking Skin

The foundation of your beauty comes from the skin. If your skin is dry, cracked or otherwise injured, chances are good that it will show in your skin no matter how much make up you put on. One way to improve the quality and look of your skin is to use a quality product designed to do so. The other way, which may be best, is to eat foods that can do much of the work for you. The food you eat is a direct reflection of what your skin looks like. The question is, then, which foods should you be eating to have great looking skin?

First, choose foods that are full of antioxidants. You want to ensure that these foods are in your diet because they keep skin looking healthy. They even work very well at aiding in improving the quality of your skin as you age. Choose foods that can do this for you. For example, to get Vitamin A, eat dairy. For Vitamin B, look to bananas, red meat and wheat germ. For Vitamin C, look to peppers, kiwi fruit, tomatoes and oranges. For Zinc, choose foods like seafood, eggs, cheese and mushrooms. Iron is also important. You can get this from red meats and seafood.

Next, consider the moisture level in your skin. If your skin is dry, you may need more essential fatty acids. Don't worry. These are not products that have a lot of grease in them. Rather, they have natural, necessary fatty oils that your body needs. You can get Omega 3 and Omega 6 oils from foods like salmon, tuna, and nuts.

Work to eat more of the deeper colors of fruits and vegetables in your diet. This makes it much easier for you to get the antioxidants you need without having to count grams. Also, keep in mind that a diet that is rich in these nutrients may feel hard to come by. When this is the case, don't be worried about using supplements. A number of supplement combinations are on the market containing all of the nutrients listed above. They can aid you in improving the quality of your skin.

When it comes to having fantastic looking skin, don't forget these very important products. You definitely need foods to be part of your health regimen for improving your skin. Otherwise, no product you add will do enough to give your skin the youth you are hoping for.

How To Have Great Eyebrows

You may not notice them often but your eyebrows really do make a statement about you. They show off your eyes and help to accentuate your overall looks. When you take the time to have great looking eyebrows, the end result is a face that is well made and well groomed. It does not have to be difficult to have great looking eyebrows like this, either.

When should you pluck your eyebrows? Does it matter? In fact it does matter. Eyebrows that are plucked should be plucked right before you go to bed. This allows for the redness caused by the plucking to fade overnight. In the morning, you will have great looking eyebrows without any swelling or redness.

Here are some more tips and hints to having great looking eyebrows:

• If you have never done your eyebrows yourself, talk with your beautician first. Not only will they do it for you, but they can help teach you how to do it. This way, you know how to shape them and how to pluck them.

• Be sure to use the right tools for the process. Purchase a pair of slant edge tweezers to aid you. These work well because they can easily grab your hair. Plus, you will need a small comb. Prior to doing any plucking, comb all of the eyebrow hair in one direction. This helps to separate them so that you can easily remove them.

• Clean up after you have finished. You will need to look just outside the normal row of hairs for your eyebrows. There may be stray pieces hiding to remove. Also, in between your two eyebrows needs to be cleaned up. Pluck any stray hairs in this region.

• Don't overdo it. You can over pluck your eyebrows. This especially is possible if you haven't taken the steps to play which hairs to pluck and have just kept working to try and even the brows out. Instead, use an eye pencil first to draw out where you want to trim and remove. This way, you are less likely to over pluck.

Taking care of your eyebrows does not need to be difficult. In fact, if you just invest a few minutes after or before you wash your face each night, chances are good you will have a great look regularly.

Eyebrows, often forgotten, but they do not have to be.

Go Organic With Make Up

You know the importance of having great looking skin. Now, why not take that to the next level by considering organic make up products. The better department stores are now getting more requests for these products and there is a reason for it. Organic products do not contain products or materials that have harmful toxins, pesticides or other non natural elements in them. In short, they are better for your skin and they are better for the environment.

Many products are now available in organic form. The more products you use that are organic, the better off you will be. Some products you are likely to find that are organic include the following items:

• Concealer and foundation products: perhaps the most important of the bunch

• Lipsticks in all shades, qualities and styles

• Blush: No limit to the colors or types either

• Eye liner: you wouldn't believe the stuff you were putting so close to your eyes

• Lotions ad topical items: these are important. Anything that you put onto your skin will get right into your pores and that ends up in your blood stream.

• Soaps and Shampoos: These are becoming more readily available by top manufacturers as organic products.

Many of the top manufacturers are providing more organic products each year. They understand the importance of this quality and they know there is a growing request for such products.

When purchasing products that are labeled organic, what should you expect? First, you should expect that the product is made up of only natural products. This means that no dyes or perfumes are used. This also means the product does not have any preservatives in them and no colorants.

They do not necessarily have to be limited in color and style, though. Many products are just as vibrant and beautiful as ever. In addition, most of these products still apply in the same format and they have a design to be high quality make up products.

When you head out to purchase the next batch of make up for yourself, why not consider purchasing products that are better for you? Choose all organic products. If you are not too sure if you will like them, purchase an organic foundation (if you use foundation.) What you are likely to find is that these products are just as high in quality, if not more so, and they go on well. You get all the same benefits without the carbon footprint.

Is Aloe Vera A Good Option?

Many people grew up with an aloe plant in their homes. They broke off the stem, a thick, spine like plant that had a number of different prickly areas on it. They felt the soft, cool liquid that oozed from it. This is aloe vera and it is one of the best products for your skin. It is all natural. It is an easy substance to get a hold of today, too, since it is readily available in many products. This is also a great way to improve the quality of your skin.

You can purchase aloe vera in a variety of forms. It is often available sold as a natural cream (look at the ingredients list to ensure it is all natural, though.) You may also find it in various medical products, such as medicated creams for dry skin. In all situations, it can provide the level of protection your skin needs from the cold weather, from dry skin or to help sooth irritation. Look at these methods to using aloe vera.

• Use it as a medication to treat the skin problems you have. It can greatly aid in improving the symptoms of someone that has eczema or psoriasis. It can also be very helpful for those who have regularly dry skin.

• Apply aloe vera to burns. It has natural soothing ability that will cool and calm the inflammation from any type of burn. It can aid in a faster recovery from those burns, too.

• Aloe Vera is a fantastic product to apply to infections like fungal infections. This includes ringworm. When it is applied, it will naturally fight off the infection, aiding your body's immune system to improve.

• You can use an Aloe Vera fluid form of medication. You can find this to be a great choice for those who need aid in reducing pain. It can also be used to aid in heartburn, ulcers, and irritable bowel syndrome.

• Use it as a product to improve skin quality. In a fluid form, it can be used in shampoos, in soaps, and in sunscreens. It is often in make up as a natural way of adding moisture to the skin.

As you can see, for anyone that is considering their beauty regimen, Aloe Vera should be a part of it. This all natural product is an all natural healer for many areas of the body. It can aid many in improving skin quality.

Your Teeth Matter

The first time that you meet someone, one of the most common things you will notice is their teeth. Their teeth are most definitely part of the process of looking good, but d you know what you should be doing to help encourage healthy teeth that look great? If not, you will want to make this your focus of your beauty regimen. Without healthy teeth, chances are good that all of the work you have done to improve your eyes and overall make up will be for nothing.

There are several things you can do today to see great looking teeth. Here are some things to take into consideration.

1. Get to your dentist. What you really need is to get to see your dentist. They will ensure your teeth are healthy and you can get a cleaning. This will spruce up your smile considerably. It can also cut down on your bad breath, which is actually a direct indication of poor teeth health.

2. Consider whitening products carefully. The whitening products that came out a few years back have been improved. They are less risky to your teeth and many of them are more effective. If you choose to purchase over the counter products, use them only as directed as over use can weaken your teeth's protective shell. On the other hand, some of the best teeth whitening are actually done right at your dentist's office. This is perhaps one of the best places to have the procedure done.

3.   Brush and floss after meals. This seems like something you have heard before, but the fact is, just one small piece of food

stuck in your teeth will make people really react poorly to you. It spoils your look! Instead, simply brush more often.

4. Consider veneers or other cosmetic procedures to help cover over your teeth or improve your smile if you have chipped, misshapen or missing teeth. The procedures can do a great deal to improve the overall look.

5. Tackle gum problems. Gums are an important part of a healthy smile. Be sure that your gums are healthy by being sure that you visit your dentist.

Your teeth really do define our overall teeth quality. Take into consideration your teeth health but also take steps to improve your smile. The good news is that if you have a great looking smile, you are more likely to smile more often.

Do Anti Aging Products Work?

When it comes to anti aging, everyone would like their skin to look the same as it did when they were in the teens and early twenties. Yet, there is no doubt that as you grow older your skin will change and with that change often comes a natural aging process. As your skin gets older, it loses some of its moisture. It also becomes less full because the natural collagen in your face starts to lesson. Over all, it is unlikely to see your skin remain perfect. Yet, there are things you can do to enable yourself to have young looking skin throughout your life.

Eat It Healthy

A good place to start is with a good diet. Believe it or not, this is one of the most powerful tools you have when it comes to improving your health. You absolutely must take the time to improve your diet if you want to have healthy looking skin for the long term. For example, you will want to include as many antioxidant rich foods possible. These foods literally keep your skin cells healthy looking because they remove dead cells and they help to keep the waste products out of the cells. This aids in keeping the skin cells flush and with as much moisture as they need.

Use Sunscreen

One of the worst things for skin is the sun. To have great looking skin as you age, you will want to ensure you are using cosmetic products that are UV protection. Your foundations should have some protection if you are not wearing any UV protection under it. The sun causes skin cancer, too, which is one of the most high risk cancers today. Even if not, up to 80 percent of the aging of your skin is from the sun.

Stop Smoking

If you stop smoking, you will see an improvement in your skin's quality. Be sure to do so as soon as possible too. When you stop smoking, it may take a few years to see any real improvement.

What else can you do to help your skin look great even as you get older? Be sure to keep yourself hydrated with at least eight glasses of water a day. Use quality make-up products, especially those that are natural. And, try yoga or meditation. Unbelievably, this holistic approach can aid your skin in looking fantastic for years to come.

Keeping Skin Hydrated Matters

Your skin is the foundation of your beauty. If you want to have skin that is amazingly beautiful, you will need to start with ensuring that you skin is hydrated. Consider a plant. When the plant's leaves get dry, they start to crack and they show their age. The good news is that even with plants, nice the leaves are fully hydrated and are regularly hydrated, they will start to get a deep green color and look full of life. The same is true for your skin. No matter what it looks like today, it can likely have improvement through hydration.

There are many ways to build up this hydrated look. What many people do not realize, though, is that the process starts with drinking enough water. Your body needs a constant supply of quality water to keep each of the cells in your body hydrated properly. Drinking other products, including juices and soda can hurt your skin. While they are fluids, they are not giving your cells enough hydration. You need water.

In addition to this, there are other ways to keep your skin hydrated. For example, during the cold winter months, the cold air can be killer on drying out your skin. Instead of allowing this to happen, apply a moisturizer to any exposed skin. This can help to lock in the hydration so that you are less likely to be hurt by the intense temperatures.

Next, consider a hydrating mist. These can be found at most good beauty salons and department stores. You simply need to spray the mist on and you will, without a doubt, have a more hydrated look. Keep in mind that it takes a good deal of time to improve skin this way. Use the other methods first, and then use this hydrating mist as a way to keep your skin looking good.

Finally, don't layer on the makeup. Your skin does need to breath. Choose make up products that are organic or at least made up of products that are not harmful to your skin. Some make up products can dry out the skin themselves.

When choosing anything that has to do with your skin, from make up to the sun screen you put on, always keep in mind the actual effect it will have on your skin. You never want a product that will draw out the moisture from your skin but instead, you do want those that lock it in.

Long Nails: Healthy Or Not So Much?

Have you thought about having long nails? Do you love the idea of having gloriously long finger nails that really make a statement when you polish them with red? When it comes to having long nails, be careful. What you might want to take into consideration is just what it means to have long nails and if this is the right type of length for you.

Why Is It Bad?

Long nails do look great, but be careful with how long you allow them to get. As your nails lengthen, there is no immediate risk to you or the nail. But, be careful about the actual length you allow. The longer the nails get, the more likely they are to be places where infectious bacteria can hide. Nails that are an inch long are more likely to have pathogens that can cause illnesses like staph infections and yeast infections.

How To Fix The Problem

If you are like most, you do not think about what is lurking under the nails. But, you should. The good news is that you can do something about it. You can have long nails and still have healthy nails. The key is to keep them clean. Use soap and a nail brush on your nails at least once a day (wash your hands using soap frequently.) The nail brush is quite effective at getting under the nails and removing all of the bacteria underneath if you take your time with it. Do not rush through the process.

Throughout the day, you can use antibacterial lotions, too. Apply these gels on your hands and also on your nails. Use them sparingly because they can dry out your nail beds and this can lead to cuts that will be even more prone to bacteria growth.

If your nails are showing any signs of illness or bacteria, trim them back. This includes any yellowing that you see. If the nail infection seems to worsen, seek out your doctor. They can prescribe medications for you that will clear up the nail beds effectively.

Having long nails is a bit more work than trimming them. Even if you have fake nails, you still need to follow these procedures to ensure that your nails remain healthy and free from any bacteria or infectious pathogens. After all, just think of all the things you do with those nails on a daily basis that could leave you sick.

CHAPTER 3- WITH BEAUTY COMES CONFIDENCE

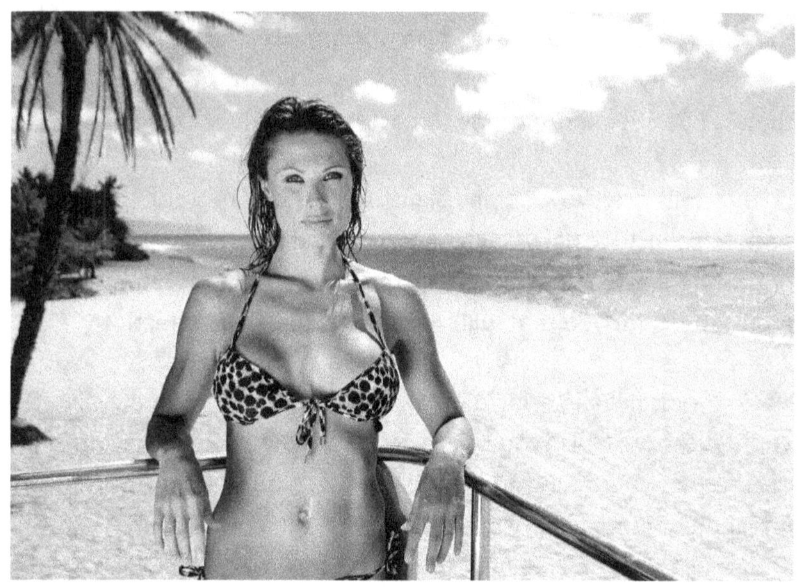

Are you looking for those movie star length eye lashes? The ones that are nothing short of truly impressive? You can get these by just making a few important decisions about the products you use and the application methods to use. Depending on how elegant you may want to be, choose the right products and do take the time to go the extra step.

Start with an eyelash curler. Use it as often as you need to, but do not overwork the lash with it. You want to be sure to use it whenever it is possible to do so. These curlers are very inexpensive but the look they give you is much appreciated. They help to make your eyes look wider and they help to give you that more alert look. For many, they can add an air of youthfulness. When you are choosing the items for your eyelashes, do not skip this step. You should only curl your eyelashes prior to applying mascara to them.

To use the eye lash curler best, place it under the hair dryer for about thirty seconds. This heats it nicely and allows it to work better with the curling. It will work much more likely a curling iron and will curl the lashes more permanently. Curl each set of lashes once. If you want a more rounded look to them, curl them twice.

Use a small comb to come through the eyelashes next. This allows them to each be separated and easy to work with. Apply a very light amount of powder to the eye lashes. You can do this using the comb. This will help the mascara to stick to the eye lashes better and this means a better look.

When applying mascara, do so with a nice, clean brush. If the brush has clumps in it, the eye lashes will also have clumps when you apply the make up to them. Place the mascara brush at the very base of your eyes and without holding it there, pull up. Applying the make up in one swoop like this is what will make it the most successful. It is important to consider a second coat, especially if your eyelashes are smaller.

Using the products you have and using them wisely will give you that great look you are hoping for. Eyelashes are an important part of overall beauty and can help to bring out your eyes.

Pick a Dominant Feature

When it comes to beauty and looking your best, one of the worst, most out of date looks you can have is a face full of makeup. Bright blue eye shadow is only second to the bright red lipstick and the amount of blush on your checks makes you look like someone has slapped you. Instead of making this mistake, you may want to try a different beauty secret. Just choose one main focal feature in your face to concentrate on. Doing so will enable everything else to glow, too.

One of the most popular options is the eyes. For those that think their eyes are their best feature, show them off. Use eye liner, eye lash mascara, and be sure to use the right eye shadow. It is find to use whatever color you would like and you most definitely will look great if you choose colors that blend well with your skin. If you choose the eyes, all of the rest of your make up should be less bright.

Perhaps your lips are your best feature. If so, use a brighter color on them and be sure to help them to stand out by using lip liner. Gloss them too, you want them to stand out and really sing your praises.

Perhaps it is not your eyes or your lips that you are most happy with in terms of your facial features. It may be your check bones. Use blush to help show off this look. You will want to use a sweeping motion, starting at the top of your check and swooping down. This really draws attention to this area of the face.

When you take the time to choose just one type of makeup application area to concentrate on, you surprisingly do not let the rest fall out of line. Rather, an individual first notices that feature, for example the eyes. They are drawn to them because of the well designed make up on them. At the same time, they are attracted to the rest of your face naturally since they have found your eyes to be appealing.

Less is more in today's make up world, but applying a concentration of make up to just certain areas of your face can make a nice statement and really helps to create that overall great look you are hoping for. Be sure to invest in quality products and a well-made face.

Sensitive Skin Can Be Maintained

There are many reasons why you may have sensitive skin. If you have spoken to your doctor and they have tackled the underlying cause, such as eczema or other skin conditions, that is great. Next, consider what make up and beauty products you can use with your sensitive skin. You will need to choose products that will not clog pores and those products that are designed specifically for individuals who have sensitive skin. There are many great products to choose.

When choosing any type of sensitive skin product, one of the first things to look for is a hypoallergenic product. This means that the product has ingredients within it that have been tested and there are no elements of it that are doing to cause an allergic reaction. Many people who have an outbreak to a product are actually having a very mild allergic reaction to the product. These hypoallergenic products are a good investment for individuals with skin that is sensitive.

Next, consider you products carefully for fragrance. Many companies add in a scent to help the product to look and smell more attractive. The problem is, though that this scent can be an instant problem for individuals who have sensitive skin.

You can find a variety of products on the market that are naturally scented or that do not have an additional ingredients added to them to add a scent. These are some of the best products for those who are suffering from conditions like peeling, eczema, dermatitis or who have allergic reactions to products.

In addition to this, you also want to choose a product that is not going to clog your pores. Your pores are the skin's tool to breathing and to taking in nutrients in some cases. They need to remain open. If and when a foundation or other make up product clogs them closed, the skin will react negatively to this situation. This can lead to pain, itching and overall breakouts on the skin.

For those who are looking for quality products that meet these specific requirements, do not skimp on value. You want to spend a bit more and buy products that will not hurt your skin. When you do so you will see improvements in the way your skin reacts when you place make up on. Look for all natural products designed specifically for individuals who have sensitive skin for the best results possible.

Stretch Marks

Perhaps you have just had a baby and you hate the stretch marks that being pregnant caused. There are other times in life when you will deal with stretch marks too. They can happen during puberty. They can also occur if you are overweight.

Stretch marks are the body's way of handling the extra size of the region. For most people, these stretched out skin marks are only temporary since as soon as the extra weight is loss, the marks become very difficult to see, if at all. Yet, for others they stick around

What Are They?

Stretch marks happen whenever the skin is over stretched. This causes the surface of the skin to be unable to develop the natural, normal amounts of collagen in the region. What happens then is that the skin simply gets a scar from the result. In medical terminology, this is called vegetures or sometimes striae.

They are generally purple in color or red in some cases. Often times they will be a less bright color especially if they have been in place for some time. Often times, they are soft and are generally noticeable just as a scar would be.

Overcoming Them

If you have stretch marks, you likely would like to do anything possible to get rid of them. The first step is to lose the weight and to do it well. In other words, you'll need to work out and tone this area of your body considerably. You can use a product like cocoa butter applied to the area. Also, dermabrasion is an option.

These methods can be highly helpful in improving the overall look of the skin. For those that have lost the weight and are unable to get the stretch marks to fade, another option is to use a laser treatment. The laser treatment allows for the removal of the damaged skin, at a very low level and allows healthy skin to heal over it.

There is no guarantee that you can get rid of the stretch marks, though. You may be able to avoid them by applying essential oils to the skin where they are beginning to show. Many times, they will fade on their own as you age. This is especially true of those stretch marks that develop during puberty. In addition to this, keep in mind that they often happen in areas of the body that are naturally covered.

Sunless Tanning: Good Or Bad?

A sunless tan is one of the best ways to avoid the harmful rays of the sun. But, are all of these products a good choice? Some are not. Some are likely to cause you to deal with all sorts of complications and skin conditions, especially if you have sensitive skin. The tanning bed is not the only option you have to have that deep, dark tan you crave. In fact, you may be able to get a better tan by simply looking around for some natural products or other alternatives.

Don't worry; you do not have to have that orange glow that many of the first products used to produce. Today's products are a better quality and for that they also work very well to produce a natural type of tan. Some o the best bronzer products are available that add a great deal of color to your skin, but the coloring is more normal looking. When choosing these over the counter bronzers, look closely at them.

Choose a product that offers a nice tan without the risk of over doing it. You also want to choose a natural bronzer if it is possible to do so. At the very least, you will need a product that contains a moisturizer in it to aid in the skin's ability to have protection from the products.

The other popular option when it comes to choosing a sunless tan option is to use a spray tan booth. These work quite simply. You will walk into the booth, activate the spray and stand still. It sprays both your front and your back for you, giving you an even tan that s very natural looking. This is a fantastic option for those who are hoping for a fast tan that is still good for them.

When choosing any sunless tanning product or spray, be sure that the product is safe o use. You not a quality product otherwise you will get results you are not happy with. In addition to this, exfoliate your skin before you apply the sunless tanning product.

This gives your skin a better finished result and will help enable the skin to pick up more of the color. When it comes to getting a tan, you definitely want one, but there is no longer a risk to your skin.

Just get out here and allow the tan from a sunless product to work for you.

Teens Beauty Tips

As a teenager, you are likely spending at least a few minutes each morning making sure you look the best. Teens have the advantage of having young, healthy looking skin. You likely do not need cover up.

You also do not likely need to spend a great deal on anti aging products. But, there are some areas that a teen may be able to improve on if she wants to have great looking skin and a good make up look that will impress anyone. No matter what your age, you can benefit from a few of these teen beauty tips.

Here are a few teen beauty tips to keep in mind.

1. Use the right type of facial cleaner. Bar soap and other soaps that are meant for hands are not good options for the face as they can be too harsh. Instead, choose a facial soap. And, be sure to remove make up each night. This step alone will keep your skin healthy.

2. Exfoliate your skin. Exfoliation is the process of using a semi abrasive product to remove some of the dead skin cells found in your pores. This helps open up those pores. It also can help to give your skin that fresh glow you are hoping.

3. Less is more with makeup. Don't believe that each of your major features on your face should stand out. Rather, just pick one major feature to stand out, such as your lips or your eyes. Use subtle make up the rest of the face. This gives you a great look without overdoing it.

4. Look for healthy products. Choose organic make up products whenever it is possible to do so. These are better for your skin and they reduce your carbon footprint.

5. Treat acne. Acne for a teen is one of the worst conditions possible. It is essential to take into consideration the variety of products on the market. What is most important is to keep your skin clean to reduce the amount of acne present. In addition to this, you should keep in mind that you will need to consider medications if your acne is severe.

Taking care f your skin as a teen will allow you to have great looking skin for years to come. Be sure to spend time working on improving the quality of your skin each day. Keep it out of the sun and be sure o use the best products you can to avoid allergic reactions.

What About Acne?

Teenagers are often plagued with acne and, most often, through no fault of their own, they have to deal with this incredibly painful and emotionally scaring type of skin condition. The problem is, for many people, acne does not go away once you hit your 20's. It can even follow you into your 30's. Acne in this case may need a bit more help than those that are simply teenage year acnes. The good news is that there is help for any type of situation.

First, start with a good cleansing regimen. Since acne is caused by the bacteria that land on your skin and imbed themselves there, a good quality cleansing will help to minimize the outbreaks. The bacteria like skin that is warm and has fatty oils in them. Plus, they love to eat the dead skin cells from your face. Cleaning with quality soap will aid in improving the acne right away. In addition to this, exfoliate. This can help to remove that dead skin which allows bacteria to grow on it. It is incredibly important to consider exfoliating properly, as you do not want to injury your face in the process.

In addition to cleansing your skin properly, be sure to take time to get extra help, if you need it. For those who have serious acne problems, seek out a dermatologist. There are medications that can aid in improving the acne problem at the source.

They can work to turn off the skin's immune system which is working so hard to kill off the bacteria (and often is what causes the acne to become so red and noticeable.) In addition to this, you want to focus on proper care for these infections. Because acne are each a small infection, it can endanger your overall health if they continue to spread. Your dermatologist can offer help in this process.

When it comes to improving your overall quality of life, acne is an important step. Applying make up to cover up the acne does not often provide enough aid to your skin. You really do need to consider removing the acne properly to help avoid the overall pain and scaring that is possible from it. Working with your dermatologist, come up with a regimen to minimize the skin's acne risk and work to improve any scars that you may have. There are wide ranges of products on the market that can aid you in this process, but your doctor should be your first step.

Chapter 4- Beauty From the Inside

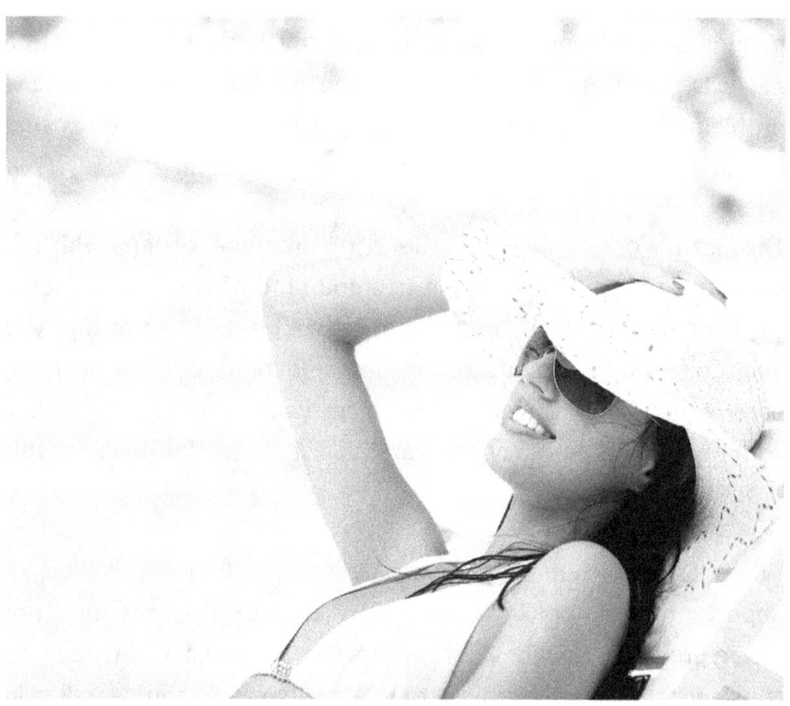

We've all heard the old saying "beauty comes from the inside" and There is a lot of truth to that statement! However, as you probably already know there are things that we can do to help enhance our natural beauty on the outside as well. In this first chapter we are going to go over a few general tips that you can use for all over beauty.

- Get plenty of sleep

To help keep yourself looking Young and beautiful be sure that you get an adequate amount of sleep every night. Never underestimate the effect that too little sleep can have on your body because it can literally age you. The average person needs from six to eight hours of sleep a night to rejuvenate their body, skin, and brain.

- Break out the baking soda

Baking soda can be your best friend when it comes to staying beautiful. It is one of those products that you should always keep handy. For beauty purposes you can use it to make your shampoo work better, especially if you have light colored hair because it will remove any residue left behind by chlorine or other things. You can also use it to whiten your teeth, take the pain of sunburn away and the best part is all this can be done for around a dollar.

- Pamper your feet

To keep your feet looking beautiful, especially during the warmer, dryer summer months, try applying Vaseline to them daily. Make sure to deeply massage it into your feet. It will keep your feet smooth and soft. Then go treat yourself to a pedicure and get a pair of strappy, sassy sandals, and show of your cute, new pedicure. With this trick you'll have the best looking feet of the season!

- Reduce the shine

If you have skin that tends to get oily and shiny, you can do one of two things throughout the day. If you want to be fancy, you can buy a packet of face-blotting sheets. These smell wonderful and are impregnated with scented transparent powder. Or you can take a sheet of regular toilet paper and press, not rub, on the oily areas. Another option is to buy a face wash that keeps your skin from getting oily and shiny.

- Extend the life of your eye shadow

Make any eye shadow bend to your will. If you are bored with the shadow choices in your everyday makeup palette, it is definitely time to spice it up a bit and get creative. Try using a moistened eye shadow brush to apply your shadow. This will give the eye shadow more pigmentation in its color and it will be brighter and more interesting than it was before. You can also use try this trick out as eyeliner!

- Switch to a pencil

Try using an eye pencil instead of liquid eyeliner if you can. Eye pencils can give a more natural subtle look, while liquid eyeliner may be too much. If you do like to use liquid liners try using an eye-lining marker. Eye markers allow you to have more control and you can do thicker, more dramatic lines, or thinner, subtle lines. If you choose to use liquid eyeliners or with any kind of eyeliner, try this trick: Pull your eyelid downward with one hand while applying the liner with your other hand.

Start from the outer corner of your eye and go towards your inner corner.

This will cause less wrinkles on your eyelids.

- Remove makeup properly

It is important that you buy a special make-up remover. Especially if you use waterproof make-up. Seeing that it is waterproof, it is much harder to remove than regular make-up and requires more than just water. If you do not have makeup remover strong enough to take off waterproof eye makeup try using some Vaseline and just massage it onto your eye then just wipe it off. I suggest using an old wash cloth to wipe the makeup off because it will stain. It is important that you remove your make-up before bed. Especially remove you foundation everyday because it will clog your pores and cause acne.

- Don't forget the SPF

Apply a lotion or cream containing SPF every day before doing your daily foundation routine. You can also purchase a tinted moisturizer. This will leave you with smooth skin and protection from the sun! You have to live your whole life with the same skin and it is worth the investment to protect it. You should definitely start off each day with a coat of sunscreen before you even think of going outside. Your skin will thank you.

- Soften while you shave

If you run out of your favorite shaving cream and you don't want to use soap to shave your legs because of the drying effect, try using hair conditioner! Coating your legs with conditioner before shaving will soften the small hairs and make it easier to shave This will leave your legs feeling super soft and silky.

While these are all great tips that you can use in your everyday life to help yourself look and feel more beautiful, the bottom line is, if you feel good about yourself then you will always be your most beautiful you!

Age with Beauty

Aging is a natural process that affects us all and as we get older most of us wishes we could slow down the effect that age has on our bodies. Even though it may not seem so our skin is very delicate and extremely sensitive to sun damage, strong chemicals, products and cosmetics.

That's why it's extremely important to protect it, treat it well and look for natural ways to help prevent damage and slow down the aging process.

Beauty Essentials for Her

There are many natural remedies and products available that can help slow down the aging process. These natural remedies are often less expensive and safer when compared to other more invasive techniques like cosmetic procedures, surgery or other chemical solutions. Which makes them a great option when it comes to reducing the effect that time has on our skin?

Generally, these more gentle treatments are composed of various natural ingredients like fruits, vegetables, botanical oils, vitamins and herbal extracts which are essential for restoring moisture, balance and restoring the elasticity of the skin while maintaining its softness, which in turn helps you maintain a younger appearance.

These herbal extracts and natural ingredients are inexpensive and can be found at your local grocery or health food store. They often provide a much better solution to cleansing and treatment than the harsh chemicals found in most over-the-counter products.

 Now let's go over a few great natural ingredients that you probably already have in your kitchen that you can use to start fighting the aging process right away:

- Coconut hydrates and moisturizes. It can be used on your skin and hair. For your skin simply grate a raw coconut, squeeze the coconut shreds, extract milk and apply the milk on the face and let it dry. Rinse it with warm water.

- Avocado is Mother Nature's moisturizer, simply mash up an avocado and apply it to your face as a mask for 15-20 minutes.

- Apply castor oil to soften your skin and eliminate wrinkles.

- Blemishes and aging spots can be removed by applying a few drops of lemon juice on the face.

- Your skin is an organ so remember to drink plenty of water to help flush away toxins and excess debris.

- Make a paste of sugar cane juice mixed with turmeric powder which is quite effective in controlling wrinkles and preventing the skin from aging.

- The enzyme in pineapple helps remove dead skin and reduces subtle signs of aging. Mash some pineapple and rub it on your face as a mask. Allow your face to dry for 10-15 minutes then rinse thoroughly.

- Certain essential oils act as effective natural remedies for anti aging. Drops of oils like sandalwood, geranium, rosewood, rose jasmine, neroli, and frankincense are to be taken and mixed with primrose oil or any other oil which can be used as base oil.

- Facial massage is another good natural remedy for anti aging. Blood circulation is increased by massage which results in tightening of the muscles and tissues.

- Green seedless grapes can be taken and cut into half and then gently crushed on the skin. Leave it for 20 minutes and then rinse it with warm water.

- Vitamin E oil or cod liver oil is to be applied daily to the skin. The aging spots shall fade.

- Remember healthy on the inside reflects on the outside so be sure and include plenty of fruits and vegetables in your diet. There are many fruits and vegetables that you can eat to help prevent aging. Some of them are carrots, cabbage, spinach, broccoli, strawberries, tomatoes, red peppers, oranges, grapes, turnips, etc.

By replacing some of the harsh chemicals that we use with more natural remedies and treatments we can all protect and nourish our bodies as well as help reduce the signs of aging on our skin.

Make Skin Radiant

If it is, then chances are you will try just about anything that promises to help make your skin have that healthy glow we all long for. Having beautiful healthy skin doesn't have to be that hard. It also doesn't require spending a fortune on over-the-counter products, treatments and serums that promise to banish wrinkles, dark spots, acne and other imperfections overnight.

Today were going to go over some simple and easy tips that you can use to help you get the healthy, beautiful and glowing skin you desire:

- Avoid wearing excess makeup and when you do make sure that you cleanse your face thoroughly afterwards. Always avoid leaving makeup on overnight!

- Always use a sunscreen and protect your skin when you go out in the sun. Even on those days that are overcast and cloudy the sun's rays can still do damage to your sensitive skin.

- Don't forget to protect your lips by using chap-stick or a lip balm with SPF protection.

- Wash your face with warm water and a gentle cleanser at least once a day. Be sure to avoid over scrubbing your skin, because it can cause it to over produce oils, which can lead to breakouts and other unwanted side effects. Cleansing helps eliminate dust and debris from your face by cleaning the pores and promoting good circulation.

- Use a good moisturizer to protect the skin from dryness. To avoid the need for two separate products look for a moisturizer with SPF protection. One of the best times to apply moisturizer is after a bath as it blocks the moisture of your skin.

- Water is essential for hydrating your skin, so as we discussed in your last issue always be sure to drink at least eight glasses of water every day. When you start following this simple tip you will see an almost immediate improvement in the quality of your skin. Plus drinking plenty of water is helpful for flushing toxins out of the body and in keeping the complexion clear and glowing.

- Get plenty of sleep. Lack of sleep reeks havoc on every part of our body, including your skin. It can lead to premature wrinkles, dry flaky patches, breakouts and more.

- A healthy and balanced diet is extremely in important to beautiful, glowing skin. a healthy diet should consist of fresh fruits and vegetables.

- Exercise regularly. By following a regular exercise program you can stimulate the blood flow to your entire body which in turn helps your skin look healthier.

- Mix 1/4 cup of milk, 2 table spoons of sugar, then dip a cotton ball and apply the milk all over the face and neck. Leave it for 15 to 20 minutes and then cleanse your face for a beautiful healthy glow.

- Make a paste by mixing a table spoon of Oatmeal with turmeric and sugar. Then gently massage the paste on your face. Leave it for 2 to 3 minutes and wash it off. This gives your skin a smooth and refreshed appearance.

These tips are simple and easy to follow. they are also more affordable than costly salon treatments or over-the-counter products. The road to beautiful skin doesn't have to be difficult in just need to find a routine that works best for you and follow it every day.

Chapter 5- Essential Hair Care Beauty Tips

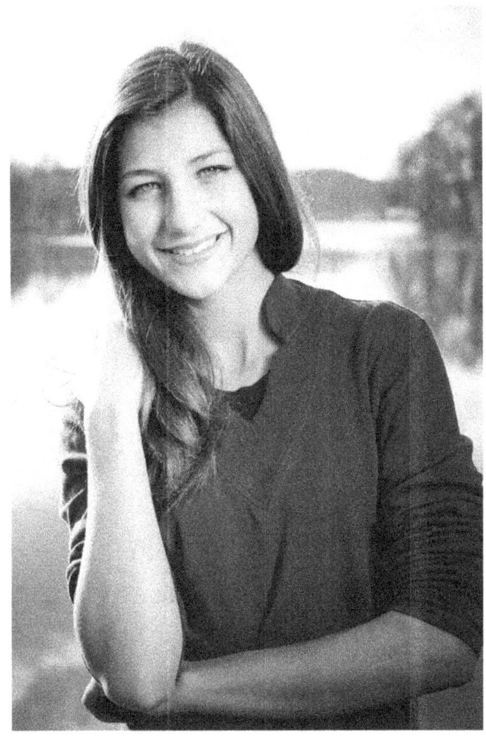

The Right Tools for the Trade

There is a tool for every job that can make life easier for you, whether it is a microwave to heat up food or the telephone to keep you in touch with the rest of the world. In the world of hair care however, there are so many products that sometimes, it is a hit or miss as to whether or not you have the right tools for your beauty regimen.

And since each person and their hair is different, what works for you may not work for someone else. So if you are a little lost in this world of hair care, listed below are some of the basics that can get you through:

Brushes and Combs

With a head of wet hair, you should never, ever use a brush of any kind, especially if you have tangles. The brushes will grab at your hair, tearing or breaking it, causing split ends and other damage.

Only a wide toothed comb will suffice. Your hair brush is an important part of your beauty routine. There are a variety of different brushes that achieve different hair styles, depending on their use.

• Bristled round brushes are often used for those with curly or wavy hair that they wish to blow dry straight.

• A paddle brush is great for every day styling and is best suited to people with long hair.

• A vented brush is great if you are in a hurry to dry your hair. They have a vented head that allows the heated air from your blow dryer to pass through the brush to dry the hair.

Hair Dryers, Curling Irons, and Straightening Tools Hair dryers have the power to fry your hair if you are not diligent about using the tool properly. The air flow should be constantly moving, rather than centering on one location. When that happens, damaged hair is the result.

Hair dryers have attachments like diffusers that will distribute the heat in a wider area to avoid damage. There are also hair dryers that use negative ion technology to cut the drying time in half and with less damage.

Curling irons and straightening tools also have the power to damage your hair. Choose these tools wisely by selecting ones that have various levels of temperature control as well as automatic shutoff mechanisms in case you forget to unplug them. For an optimal performing curling iron or straightening tool, go with those that are made with ceramic technology. Ceramic is less likely to burn your hair and it will even provide some conditioning as it heats your hair into shape.

Shampoos

Your scalp should dictate what type of shampoo you use. If you have dandruff, you would need something specific to that condition. Oily or dry hair also dictates what type of shampoo to use. You need to shampoo every time you wash your hair to get rid of the dirt and other pollutants that you might pick up in the course of your day. Be careful and try to avoid any shampoos that have any type of alcohol in the ingredients. Alcohol can dry out your hair.

Conditioners

There is some debate as to whether or not you even need conditioner. For the most part, you do, unless you have super fine hair that looks lifeless when you use a conditioner. Hair care products, brushing, drying, curling and straightening your hair can be damaging, not to mention colors or perms. A conditioner can replenish and protect your hair from these damaging elements. To avoid oily or dull looking hair on the crown of your head, only apply conditioner to the length of your hair and avoid the scalp.

Hairsprays and Other Styling Products

A few decades ago, hairsprays had the power to eat through a hole in the ozone layer. These days, they are more environmentally friendly without harsh chemicals. The hairspray of today can protect against humid conditions and even the sun's harmful UV rays. There are a variety of formulas depending on what styles you hope to achieve.

Mousses, gel and shine serums are great for those people who have problems achieve a smooth finish without compromising any bounce and body in their hair. If you have fine hair, mousses are light and work best for the hair. With thicker heads of hair, gels work the best. Shine serums are for those people who have dull looking hair, even when it is clean. Shine serums can also sometimes perform double-duty as a frizz controller.

When in doubt, talk with your stylist about what products would best suit your hair. Ask questions each time they use a different product in your hair to achieve a certain look. They can guide you through that confusing maze of hair care tools.

CHAPTER 6- ESSENTIAL SKIN CARE BEAUTY TIPS

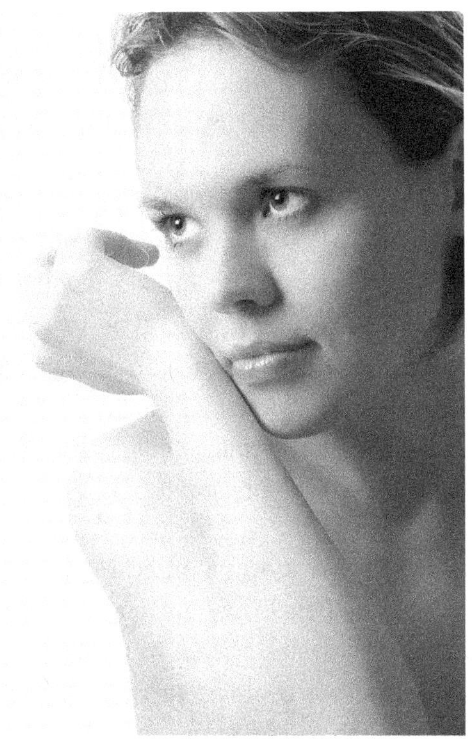

At some point in your life, you will start to reflect on your aging. It might be a line that shows up or a gray hair that catches your eye as you look in the mirror. Either way, though, you will see it and it will be time to start considering the implication of growing old. You don't want to just lie down and take it, though, do you?

The number one way you can fight the effects of aging is by taking care of your skin. By taking the proper measures to care for your skin from head to toe, you will be able to reverse some of those effects of aging while at the same time improving the health of your skin as well.

What steps should you take then? The best way to remember is that you have to keep with your "ABC's" when caring for your skin from head to toe. "A" is for anti-aging cream, "B" is for blemish control, and "C" is for collagen. If you keep those three words in mind, you will be well on your way to proper skin care and reversal of those wrinkles associated with aging. Each word is a reminder about an important step in the skin care and age reversing process.

"A" is for anti-aging cream, and that is an incredibly important step in the care of your skin. Hopefully you were properly hydrating and caring for your skin before that first wrinkle. If you weren't, though, once you see that little aging sign it is time to spring into action. Waiting or ignoring the wrinkle is the worst thing you can do. Once you see a sign at all, application of a quality anti-aging cream will possibly stop new lines from forming while getting rid of the one or two wrinkles that have shown up already.

Though anti-aging creams are not miracle drugs or fountains of youth, they do actually help. They are made up of vital vitamins and nutrients that science has proven to rejuvenate skin. Look for an anti- aging cream that contains Retinol. Retinol is a form of Vitamin A that has been shown to rejuvenate the effects of aging on the skin.

"B" is for blemish control. Blemishes, pimples, zits if you will, are not only for teenagers. They are something that can affect your skin for your entire life. So you need to always be diligent in your search for and treatment of blemishes and potential blemishes. They can manifest themselves in a number of ways: whiteheads, blackheads, and minor inflammations. Each should be caught as early as possible since they actually can be prevented in most cases. If you can't stop them, you can conceal or cure them with over the counter medications and skin care products. What you use will vary depending on when you catch the blemish and what kind it is. Just be sure to use the proper medication rather than squeezing and popping your blemishes which can cause scarring and in some cases can even lead to more blemishes down the road.

"C" is for collagen. Collagen is contained in your skin and is what makes it elastic and smooth. As you age, the collagen molecules in the skin begin to break down .This break down creates wrinkles and lines on your face and body. The problem in the past has been that anti-aging creams could only use partial collagen molecules because they are large and difficult to get into the skin through lotion.

Recently, though, one major company developed and patented an infusion system for collagen. With it, creams can deliver whole collagen molecules into the skin. Once the collagen has been delivered, there is a noticeable difference. Your skin will have a healthy and rejuvenated glow. In addition, the wrinkles and lines that come with aging will begin to dissipate. Collagen is important, and it is the closest thing we currently have to a miracle aging cure.

If you are ready to put up a fight against the effects of aging, the process is going to start with your skin. Take the time to learn you're "ABC's" of skin care and you will start to look younger and your skin will begin to feel better. Remember, anti-aging cream, blemish patrol, and collagen is the key to your fight against aging skin.

Combination Skin

Combination skin is when you have certain areas on your face that are dry and others that are oily.

Usually, the oily part of your face is in what is called the "t-zone" or the area of your forehead, nose and chin. When you have combination skin, you will probably notice that most days, you will experiences normal or dry skin. There are several ways you can take care of your combination skin. Here are six strategies for a healthy glow.

How can you be certain you have combination skin? If you have combination skin, your skin on your face might feel tight or dry after washing or taking a shower. Your face might also feel rough, look flaky or have an overall dull appearance. On the other hand, on other areas of your face, you will experience shiny skin that might feel or look greasy. This is most common in the "t-zone". Those areas are more prone to developing blackheads, pimples or other bumps.

There are ways to care for combination skin. After you have determined what kind of skin you have on your face, you can take steps to find the proper products and care for your skin. It may be that you have combination skin during certain seasons, such as summer. Your skin may be normal during other parts of the year. People, who spend a lot of time outdoors, might experience a dry skin all year round.

The first step you can take to treat and care for your combination skin is to cleanse. Look for products that are made specifically for combination skin and use it twice a day. This will help combat the oily skin on the "t-zone" and help keep other parts of the skin healthy. Make sure that you keep your face clean and free of residues at night. This is a good step to take towards caring for combination skin.

The second step to care for combination skin is to moisturize. When you have combination skin, some parts of your face might be oily, but other parts are dry and flaky. You cannot ignore the dry skin when treating the oily skin. The answer is to use moisturizer on the dry skin only. Products made for dry skin will help hydrate the dull and flaky skin. Try to keep the moisturizer off of the oily skin. That will only make it worse.

The third step is to balance your skin. There are many products that can help normalize your skin. Look for those that have alpha hydroxy acids, or retinol, which is a vitamin A product. Also, use a toner everyday to help keep the skin in balance. Steer clear of products that contain alcohol because that can irritate dry skin. Use toner at least once a week to combat combination skin.

The fourth step is to control the skin by eating healthy and drinking plenty of water. When you practice a healthy diet, you can take a big step in controlling the quality of your skin. Fatty and greasy foods are not good for any type of complexion. Eat lots of fresh fruits and vegetables and try healthier oils. Drinking water will also help by hydrating your skin the natural way.

The fifth step is to use appropriate make up. Make up that contains oil-absorbing properties will help your appearance. Oil-free make up and make up that is labeled as non-comedogenic will help by minimizing the chances to pimples and blackheads. Another important part of skin care is to make sure make up is thoroughly removed each night before bed. Never go to bed with make up on because it can cause skin irritations.

The sixth step is to use a good sunscreen. Look for sunscreens with an SPF of at least 15. Using a daily sunscreen will help ensure that your skin does not become sunburned, which leads to dry skin. There are several varieties of sunscreen that are made specifically for daily use on the face. In addition, look for moisturizers and make ups that already contain sunscreen for added benefit. Using sunscreen every day, even in the winter, will help ensure that you have a healthy glow to your skin.

Masks, Scrubs, Exfoliating Products

Your skin is the first thing that people probably notice about you. Did you know that it also plays a vital role as your body's largest organ? It protects your muscles, bones, blood vessels and internal organs. So, if the skin is so vital, why do some people not take proper care of it? Going outside without sunscreen, using harsh products and not drinking enough water and other fluids does not help matters. You have to live with your skin all your life, so why not treat it with the utmost care?

There are a countless products on the market these days that can help you achieve healthy skin. You just have to know what to do.

Before determining the best skin care regiment, you have to determine what condition or skin type you have. If you are one of the lucky few, you might have normal skin – nothing too dry or oily. A large part of the population might have combination skin where there are parts of your face and body that are dry and other parts that are oily. Or, you might just be one oily mess! No matter what skin type you might be, there are products made that cater just to you. Among these many products made for your face are facials masks, scrubs and exfoliating products. Do you have any ideas what these skin care products accomplish in your beauty care regiment? If not, then read on for some highlights:

Facial Masks

There are a variety of facial mask products that are made for any condition or skin type. If you are plagued by acne or blackheads, there are facial masks that you apply, then let dry. Once dry, you can peel them off and hopefully some dead skin covering those blackheads will become unclogged so you can clear them up. There are also facial masks, like a mud mask that you apply and allow to dry. Afterwards, you would wash your face with warm water to clean off the mud mask.

These mud masks offer a variety of benefits like oil control. You skin afterward will have a healthy glow and not be shiny from oil. The mud masks remove impurities in your skin's pores as well as minimize the appearance of those pores. Pimple production is reduced and also blackheads dissolve and wash away once you remove the mask.

Just think of exfoliating as using a piece of fine sandpaper on your skin. You are using a mildly abrasive substance which buffs the dead skin cells away, leaving healthy, glowing skin behind. There are several benefits to exfoliating. For one, the old dead skin cells that make your complexion dull are buffed away, leaving new skin cells that are vital and fresh. Secondly, after exfoliation, your skin can more readily absorb any moisturizers or other skin treatments.

There is some debate in the beauty world as to how often you should use some type of exfoliating product on your face, heck on your whole body for that matter. If your skin leans toward normal to oily skin, exfoliating is beneficial about three to four times a week. This action will also help with the excess oil production on your skin. With drier skin, exfoliation should only be done maybe once or twice a week at the most.

For facial masks and scrubs to be truly beneficial to you and your skin, you must follow a beauty routine that encompasses both of these products and more. Use cold cream or a product that matches your skin type to remove your makeup daily. Then use a light cleanser to remove any light traces of makeup. The next step would be to exfoliate. This can be a homemade remedy like a paste made from baking soda or lemon and sugar. Or, you can purchase a specially formulated salt or sugar scrub that will accomplish the same thing. From there, you would rinse off all traces of the exfoliating product, then moisturize, again using a product based on your skin type.

The facial mask is something that is best suited during a relaxing bath in place of exfoliating. They should be used once all traces of makeup are removed. If you want to minimize the appearance of wrinkles and pores, then facial masks are the way to go.

Skin care is not complicated once you know all the players involved. What is hard is being diligent about your beauty routine and not skipping a step or two. However, the rewards of younger, vibrant looking skin more than make up for those extra efforts.

CHAPTER 7- MAKE-UP BEAUTY CARE

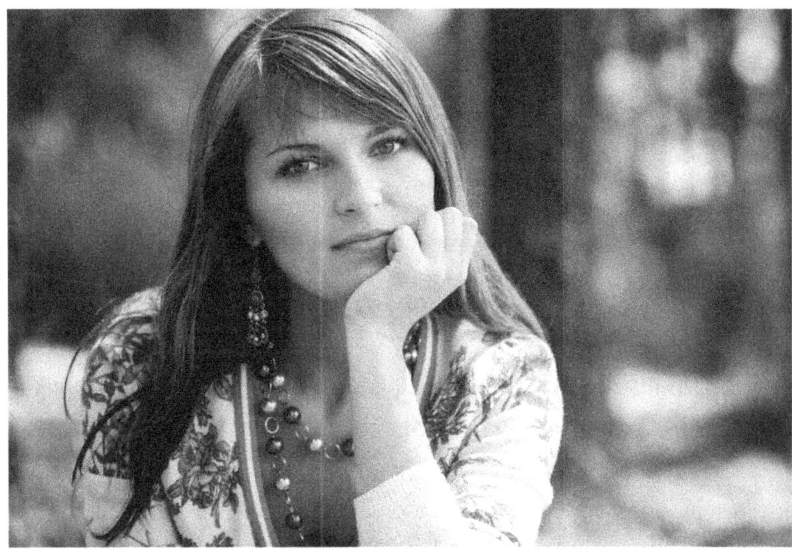

Learning the correct techniques when applying make-up can help you look your best. When you know what types of make-up to use and how to properly apply them, you can make sure your appearance is always at its best. In addition to learning how to apply makeup, you should also understand what types of products are best for your skin type and what colors are most flattering to your complexion.

Applying makeup using the correct techniques does not have to be difficult or frustrating. There are two very common mistakes that women make when they apply makeup. They either use the wrong colors, or they apply too much make up. Using the wrong colors can make anyone look like they have just been playing in their mother's make up bag.

Generally, chose colors that compliment your skin tones. If you have light skin, do not go with dark colors. Also, do not try to apply too much make up. Apply just enough for a natural glow.

When you are ready to apply makeup, consider using a concealer. Concealer can help you hide under the eye circles, or flaws and blemishes on your skin. This can enhance the overall look of your face. Look for a concealer that closely matches your skin tone. If you get a color that is too light or too dark, it will show. When you apply the concealer, do not stretch the skin. Instead use a light patting motion. Concealer comes in stick creams, bottles and powders.

After you have covered your dark circles or blemishes you will be ready to apply foundation or base. This usually comes in a thin cream and also matches the color of your skin. Not everyone uses foundation, but if you have uneven skin tone or freckles, using foundation can enhance your appearance. When apply foundation, use a makeup wedge or your fingers. Generally, start applying from your nose and work your way out. Make certain that the foundation is well blended around the edges of your face so the line is not visible.

The next step in applying makeup is to use apply blush. Blush also comes in many colors and varieties. Powder blush is probably the most popular, followed by sticks or creams. Find a shade that compliments your skin tone. If you are applying the powder variety, use an angled make up brush and apply the powder on the apples of your checks. Brush the powder upwards towards your temples.

You can then blend in the powder using another brush. Make sure the blush is well blended around the temples making sure that the fine powder is not in the hairline.

After you have applied blush, you can apply the eye makeup. Eye shadow can be a fun product to use if you want to experiment with different colors. Try shades until you find one that is flattering to you.

When applying eye shadows start at the corner of the eyelid and apply it going out. You can either use the applicator the makeup comes with or use a small brush that will look like a flat paintbrush. You can then apply a lighter shade on the top of your eyelid and blend the two colors together. You can even experiment with using several shades together as long as you blend the colors together.

Now you can apply eyeliner and mascara. When you apply eye makeup, be careful to use clean applicators and never lick the eyeliner. Do not apply eyeliner on the inside of the eyelid. Eyeliner comes in various shades and in pencil form or a liquid form.

Pencil eyeliner is usually easier to apply than the liquid. Mascara also comes in several colors. If you have droopy eyelashes, consider using an eyelash curler for maximum effect. For those that suffer from watery eyes from allergies or who swim, look into using waterproof mascara.

When you are done, you can apply your lipstick. As a general rule, do not go to bright if you have pale skin. Make sure that you thoroughly remove all make up before going to bed each night. Also, throw away old make up when it is dry or cracked. Do not try to use old or expired make up, especially around the eye area.

Foundation Facts

Everyone has their own natural beauty. And for centuries, ladies have been using makeup in some form or fashion to enhance that beauty. These days, the cosmetic industry is booming with a plethora of products from eyebrow pencils to lipsticks to eye shadows to foundation. It is foundation, or liquid makeup, that provides the base for most women's beauty regiments.

Obviously, with the variety of ethnicity and skin types, all foundations are not created equal. So how do you decide which foundation is right for you? First of all, you have to know where to buy your foundation.

You can purchase your makeup from the grocery store or even a pharmacy. And while there are some great makeup buys at those stores like eye pencils and lipsticks, the best place to buy your foundation is a department store. The makeup counters have experienced personnel who know about the various products that complement certain skin types as well as matching the skin tone and application techniques.

One of the first things you have to consider in regards to choosing the foundation that works best for you is your skin type. What condition is your skin in? Do you have dry or flaky skin? What about oily skin? Or maybe, your skin is a combination of the two. If you are a little unsure of what may describe your skin condition, ask for the opinion of the makeup consultant at the department store beauty counter.

After determining your skin type, you have to decide which foundation formula would best suit your needs. If your skin is dry, hydrating or moisturizing foundation formulas are great choices to provide a great base for you beauty regiment. Oil control foundations work best for the oily skin. And if you are prone to breakouts, look for formulas that cater to acne-free results. When you have combination skin, you need to find a foundation formula that would suit both oiliness and dryness.

When shopping for new foundation, make sure that you are not wearing makeup already. Having a clean face will ensure that you can apply a few colors of foundation on your face without it clashing with something else.

Determining your skin tone is very helpful in choosing the best foundation as the basis for your makeup. Fair skin might require a foundation with rosy undertones while a darker complexion might need something more yellow- based in color. With the multitude of skin colors – from the fair skin of Caucasians to the olive complexions of Latin descendants to the darker undertones of African Americans or Middle East Asians, there are a countless shades to choose from.

Pick the two or three shades that you think might best suit your skin tone. Apply the foundation shades at various places along your jaw line. Your skin in this area is the most true to the type of makeup color you need.

Whatever you do, do not apply the makeup on your wrist or hand because these are not optimal areas to best determine the foundation's tone and color. Because the lighting in the store is mostly fluorescent, you want to go outside in natural sunlight to look at how well the foundation blends in with your skin. Your best selection would be the one foundation that is virtually undetectable on your skin. You should be the one wearing your makeup, not the makeup wearing you.

The reason why buying your foundation at a department store is stressed is because no one person perfects fits the standards colors you may find in a pharmacy or grocery store. For the most part, people are in between shades. The department stores offer higher end foundations that are possible to custom blend into the shade you require. Another reason that department stores are optimal for your foundation purchase is because the makeup consultants can give you tips on applying your foundation as well as suggest complementary products or alternatives that you may not have thought of like concealer or tinted sunscreen or moisturizer.

Be sure and think about what you want out of your foundation as well. Do you want light and natural or something that makes your skin more luminous for evening events? How about a satiny finish or matte finish? The possibilities are many, but your needs are few. Decide what role your makeup will play in your daily life and activities and choose the best foundation that fits that role.

Don't Trowel on Makeup!

Ever get frustrated when you set out to do a task, but don't have all the proper tools to help you achieve the best possible results? Just think about that when you are applying your makeup. Having the right tools can make all the different in the world, whether you are applying makeup to conceal imperfections or highlighting your assets. So how do you know which ones would best suit your needs? And how do you know which ones that you absolutely cannot live without? Read on to find out about the six make up tool "must-haves":

1. Makeup Sponges

Many women might use their fingertips to apply their foundation. While there is no real problem with that, sponges are definitely more advantageous. First of all, if you are prone to breakouts, your fingertips might add that extra oil you skin really doesn't need. Secondly, makeup will stay on your face for more even coverage than if with the fingertips. Plus, blending is easier and less noticeable with a sponge.

Triangular shaped sponges work the best to get into the crevices of your face like around your eyes and along your nose. They are also great for blending foundation and other makeup along the jaw or hair lines without any noticeable makeup lines. Sponges can also be reused several times and even washed to prolong its usefulness.

2. Powder Brush

A thick, lush power brush is a necessity in your beauty palette of tools. Most face powders come with a small applicator or powder puff. These devices do not adequately distribute the face powder on your face. The powder brush will help blend the powder and give you control on exactly where you want the powder applied.

3. Eyebrow Brush

Your eyebrows are like the window dressing to your eyes. When your eyebrows are not groomed properly, it is one of the first things people notice. Brushing your eyebrows into a certain shape can help you identify those errant hairs that need plucking. Also, an eyebrow brush can best distribute a little color to your brows in case you have to fill in any "bald" spots or enhance the brow color.

4. Eyelash Curler

This is a tool that is not in many women's repertoire yet it has the power to really make your eyes pop. The eyelash curler is especially helpful to ladies whose lashes don't curl up very well. The trick is to briefly heat up the curler with a hair dryer, and then curl the ends of the lashes for several seconds. Once completed, you would follow up with an application of mascara to the lashes to maintain that curl.

5. Eye Shadow Sponge Applicator

Eye shadow can sometimes appear flaky upon application. The eye shadow sponge applicator allows more control over gliding the makeup along your eyelids, thus reducing the chance of powder flakes from escaping. In addition, the use of a sponge applicator allows for easier color blending, especially if you are using a base color on the lower lid along with a highlighting color above it.

6. Foundation or Concealer Brush

Many makeup artists are now swearing by using a thick, densely packed brush to apply foundation. The reasoning is that it gives you a light application of makeup without looking "made up." It is a great blending tool. Concealer brushes are similar in scope, except have a smaller head for easier manipulation for smaller areas. Even if you don't wear foundation, you can use it to apply a concealer for dark under eye circles, blemishes or other imperfections.

You can probably "get by" without these six makeup tools. However, when they are available and you add them to your beauty regiment, you will notice a discernable difference in your appearance after your makeup application. Makeup will look more natural on your skin with no noticeable delineations. You will also find that you have cut down your prep time in your beauty routine. Some of these tools can be bought at the dollar store or a pharmacy. However, if you want your beauty tools to last, consider a trip to the department store makeup counter. Sure, these makeup tools will be more expensive, but remember – you are investing in your appearance!

Aren't you worth that investment?

Blushing Basics

Some people are born with natural high cheekbones and some people need a little help in accentuating what they have. That is why having blush as part of your makeup and beauty regiment is important.

Not quite half of women these days wear blush and those that do, apply blush incorrectly. Adding blush to your makeup routine can perk up a face that appears washed out or colorless. If you are tired and decide only to apply a few beauty essentials to your face, blush should be one of those items.

Blush can give you the appearance of being wide- eyed bushy-tailed when in actuality, you are exhausted and need help getting through the day.

One of the most important questions that women have in selecting blush is what color they should get. That can be a hard task if you don't have a natural eye for color. If you don't want to subject yourself to the makeup counter at a department store, there are one or two things that can guide you to a color decision. First, think about when you exercise or do some type of strenuous activity.

Getting physical puts color in your cheeks doesn't it? The color you achieve in your cheeks from a light physical activity is one way to steer you to an appropriate blush color. Another way is to pinch your cheeks and wait a second or two. The color you get from those pinches should also help in your decision.

Your second step on the road to a beautiful blush is to decide what type of blush to purchase. There is a variety to choose from including the powder, gel, cream and tint blushes. The condition of your skin should dictate what type of blush you want to buy.

Here is a brief breakdown of each:

• Powder blushes are universal, meaning that most skin types can wear them. If you want a long-lasting color, powder blushes are the best.

• Gel blushes provide more of a translucent shine and are best suited to those oily to normal skin types. It is best applied with the fingertips and dries fast.

• Cream blushes can also be applied with the fingertips. They are thick in consistency, but not overwhelming on the skin once applied.

Because cream blushes are rich in moisturizing ingredients, they are best suited to those women with dry skin.

• Tint blushes are like a cheek stain. It dries very quickly, so you have to move fast to apply it correctly without streaks or mishaps. Tint blushes are the least user-friendly but last until you wash your face.

Now that you have an idea of the types of blushes to choose from, it is time to apply the product to your face. You want to make sure and complete most of your makeup routine first, meaning foundation, powder and any eye products like shadow, eye liner and mascara.

Blush is considered the finishing touch. If you are completely done with your other makeup, you will have a better idea of how much blush to apply.

Determine what the shape of your face might be. Knowing whether you have a round, oval, square or heart-shaped face will give you a better guide as to where the blush is going to be applied. Dip your brush or applicator into the blush and tap it to shake off the excess. Look into your mirror and smile.

You should have a hint of where your cheekbones are; the rounded part of your cheekbones is called the "apple" and that is where you need to apply the blush. Start at the "apple" and follow the natural contour of your cheekbone, toward your hairline.

Blend the color so there is no obvious delineated blush line. You want the color to look as if nature put it there.

Don't worry if you apply too much blush, especially if it is a powder blush. You can use your translucent face powder to gently blot over your blush to tone it down if need be. To get the best results, do not use the dinky blush brush that comes with your makeup. Purchase a separate, professional blush brush that you can purchase at any makeup department store counter or beauty supply store. If you want the best results, you have got to have the right tools!

Eye Makeup Tips

Your eyes are a barometer of your mood, a window into how you are feeling. Just one look can show sadness, joy, pain, happiness, exhaustion or thoughtfulness. Your eye color, whether blue, green, brown or shades in between, expresses thoughts which are not always said. That is why, for women, eye makeup is an important part of their beauty routine.

A beautifully made-up eye can enhance those come hither looks when you want to be flirtatious. If you want to appear mysterious, eye makeup can help you achieve that look as well. Expressing a mood and accentuating the eyes are among the most important reasons why women take great pains to apply their eye makeup. When adorning the eyes, you are talking about a variety of products that can be used. Eyebrow pencils, eye shadow, eyeliner and mascara are a few of the main items that are used in a beauty regiment. You can read on for some advice on eye makeup:

1. Eye Shadow

Just because eye shadows come in a palette of colors does not mean you have to go hog wild in its application. If you go for too much color you will end up looking like Bozo the Clown. The key is to choose neutral, understated colors first to get the hang of applying the makeup.

Make sure that the colors you do use complement each other. Luckily, many eye shadows come in pre- made color palettes, so you don't have to guess which color will provide a base and which one will be a highlighted color along your brow bone. Most eye shadows are in a compressed powder form and you use a foam brush for application.

There are some cream shadows however that glide effortlessly and are easy to apply with either your fingertip or a small eye shadow brush. Eye shadow pencils are also gaining popularity.

2. Eyeliner

There are numerous options when it comes to eyeliner. There is liquid eyeliner that is applied with a small brush. You need a gentle, steady hand to apply the eyeliner. There are also eyeliner pencils that you have to sharpen periodically. This option more readily defines your eyes and you have more control in its application. Some eyeliner pencils come with a built-in sponge "smudgers" that can blend in your eyeliner for a smoky, sultry look.

3. Mascara

This is a product that many women say they cannot live without. Even if they don't wear any other makeup, they wear mascara because it has the power to "wake" up and accentuate your eyes. If your lashes are pretty meager, mascara can plump them up and make you appear to have more lashes than you really do. It is important that you dab the excess mascara off the wand before applying, starting at the base, to ensure that it does not clump. There are a variety of colors and formulas. You might consider waterproof mascara if you have allergies or plan on doing any crying (like attending a wedding). It won't budge unless you wash it off.

To make your eyes really pop, there are a few tips you can try, like utilizing an eyelash curler. Use your hair dryer to briefly heat it up, and then curl your lashes. Once your lashes appear longer, with more curl, apply a mascara to set it.   A lightly sculpted eyebrow also works wonders for accentuating the eyes. Use an eyebrow brush to groom the hairs, and then pluck any errant strands.

Clean lines and a light application of eyebrow pencil will help in your quest for pretty peepers.

Taking care of under your eyes is also part of the beauty regiment. If you have circles under your eyes, you need to make sure that you get enough sleep at night and drink plenty of water to stay hydrated. Also, sometimes, it is allergies that cause dark circles under the eyes. You might have to resort to under eye concealer as camouflage.

Once you get the hang of applying eye makeup, don't be afraid to experiment a little, either with a colored eyeliner or mascara. Have a home spa makeover day with some friends and play around with a casual, light daytime look or an evening party-girl look. With a little experimentation, you could be ready for any event with a gorgeous pair of eyes that really pop.

Chapter 8- Wear a Perfect and Beautiful Smile

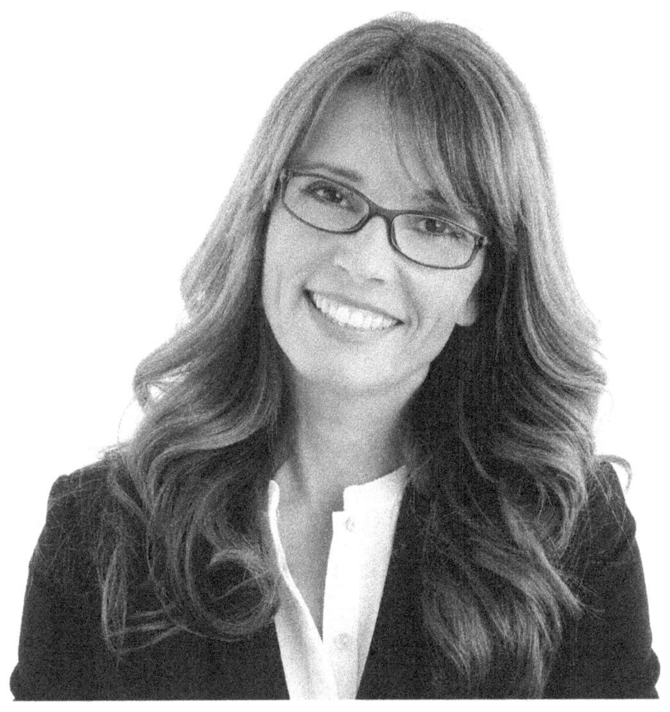

Chapped lips are painful because the dry and cracked lips are usually sore or bleeding. Chapped lips are most common in cold, windy and dry weather or when exposed to the outdoors for long periods of times. Sunburns can also cause lips to become chapped and painful. Lips are not able to produce the same types of oils that other parts of our skin do, so the result is that they become dry easily.

The natural reaction to dry lips is to lick or bite the lips. This does not help, and in fact, can make the situation worse. Severe chapped lips are flaky, bleeding and very uncomfortable. Anyone can suffer from chapped lips, including children. The key to treating chapped lips is to moisturize and treat your lips with a little respect.

The biggest thing you can do to treat and prevent dry, chapped lips is to use moisturizing chapstick. Chapstick is inexpensive and is easy to find at most retail and drugstores. Look for a chapstick that contains beeswax, phenol and sunscreen for the best results. Remember to have chapstick on hand during the whole year, not just the winter months.

Using chapstick on a regular basis will help your lips stay smooth and moist. Other types of products you can use to help chapped lips include Vitamin E and aloe vera products.

There are some types of chapstick that should be avoided. Flavored lip balms and some types of lipstick can often cause a more drying effect. Also, with children, a flavored lip balm might tempt children to lick their lips to taste the flavor. Licking will only cause the lips to become drier.

To prevent chapped lips, make sure you use a good chapstick before going outside each time. Have it in your pocket and ready for use. If you spend a good deal of time outside, especially in the winter months, reapply the chapstick several times while you are outside. This can also help prevent dry, cracked lips.

If you find yourself without chapstick and you know you need it, you can rub the side of your nose with your finger and then rub your lips. The oil from your skin will help keep your lips hydrated when you are in a pinch. If you know you will be outside for long periods of time, either use a chapstick that contains sunscreen or apply sunscreen to your lips. Sunburns will definitely affect your lips.

Another key prevention in chapped lips is to stay hydrated. That means you should drink plenty of water and fluids, especially during the hot months and the winter. When your body is dehydrated, your skin will suffer. As a result, your lips will become dry, as well. Also, you may feel a natural urge to lick your lips when your mouth feels dry and thirsty. This will cause your lips to become dry and parched.

Keep a bottle of water handy and take drinks when you feel like you are thirsty or dry.

You can also help keep your lips soft and smooth during the winter months by covering your mouth with a scarf or masks when you go outside. This is especially important for children who will not notice that their lips are becoming dry and cracked. During the winter months, you can also combat dry, chapped lips by using a humidifier at home or at work. You can sleep with a humidifier on at night and it will help keep your lips moisturized.

If you wear dentures, dry lips can be caused by improper fittings. If you suspect this is the reason for your dry lips, speak to your dentist and have the dentures refitted. The same goes for other dental devices, such as retainers, braces or dental partials. If you have poor fitting dental devices, this can cause you to breath out of your mouth. This will quickly dry out your lips causing dry, cracked lips.

In addition, getting sick is another common reason for getting dry lips. If you are suffering from a cold, be sure to take care of yourself. Use chapstick, stay hydrated and eat well. Fruits and vegetables will help keep your body hydrated and healthy during illnesses. Knowing how to prevent and treat dry, chapped lips will help you look and feel your best.

Paying Lip Service

Your lips are one of the most prominent and noticeable parts of your body, but you may not always pay attention to them the way you should. Your lips, as part of your mouth, draw attention every time you talk, smile, or even when you subconsciously lick them.
Since they do spend so much time in the eyes of people you are around, then shouldn't you make sure you are taking proper care of them? Lip care can improve your smile, your charm, and the way people view you, so it really is worth your time.

The problem most people have is that they don't really realize that lips are not the same as the other skin on your body. In fact, your lips are one of the most delicate and fragile parts of your body and should be treated as such.

They are not made up of as many layers of skin as the rest of your body is which makes them more susceptible to drying, cracking, and chapping. In addition, they do not have their own oil glands which means without assistance they are more likely to dry out than the rest of your skin. Once you have realized that your lips are different, it is time to start thinking about how you can care for them.

The number one thing you can do to care for your lips is actually good for the rest of you too. You should be hydrating yourself regularly. Drink more water and less alcohol and caffeine. If you live in a dry region, you may even want to invest in a humidifier in your home. In addition, you should be applying Chapstick and other lip balms on a regular basis. All of these things are needed to keep your lips from drying out which is the number one problem you will get since, as mentioned before, they do not produce their own oils like the rest of your skin does.

You should also continue to protect and moisturize your skin as the day goes on, with something other than saliva. This will help to condition your lips and hydrate them to prevent the damage the elements can cause. You should also be aware of what kind of lip gloss or balm you are using. Wax based balms and glosses protect your lips well, but petroleum moisturizing products correct without protecting. So you may even want to look for both.

Another tip to keep your lips looking good and feeling good is to stay away from heat. Stay away from hot showers, hot baths, and the hot sun. Hot baths and showers damage your lips by triggering dryness and taking moisture from them at the same time.

If you are going to be outside during the summer months a lot, then you should use a wax- based lip balm or lip gloss. The SPF should also be at least a 15, but preferably more to protect you from the sun. During the winter, you should also be protecting your lips from the elements that can damage them. The reflected sunlight from the snow can be very hard on your lips, so continue to protect from the sun even in the cold winter months.

Another lip care strategy is to not smoke. Smoking, as you well know, is bad for you anyway, but it is terrible for your lips. It does damage to your entire mouth which includes your lips. In addition, the smoke itself will dry out your lips and kill healthy cells on a regular basis. In addition, it can discolor your lips the same way it does your teeth. Who wants tobacco stained lips, anyway?

You lips are not only some of the most prominent and noticeable parts of your body, but they are also covered in the most sensitive skin you have. Kissing is pleasurable due to that sensitivity, but aside from that it only means that your lips require a lot of care. Stay hydrated since lips do not produce oils, don't smoke because it can damage your lips, and keep away from heat. All the while, be sure to wear a good lip balm or lip gloss to keep your lips looking good and feeling great.

Teeth Whitening Tips

Perhaps the greatest trend in dental care right now is teeth whitening. There are a number of ways you can get whiter teeth for that brighter smile. At the same time, there are just as many levels of cost associated with those methods as well as levels of risk that are connected with certain ways of teeth whitening. With varying cost levels, risk factors, and a certain amount of mystery in long-term teeth whitening effects, it makes sense to explore some of the natural methods of whitening your teeth. You don't have to resort to chemicals if you don't want to, there are other ways.

As you stroll down the dental care aisle at your local drug store or mega-mart, you will see that there are rows and rows of teeth whitening products. You will see mouth washes, gums, toothpastes, and even film treatments that you stick on your teeth for hours at a time. These are all quick fixes.

If you want to use the natural methods of teeth whitening, though, you will need to be patient. Most of the natural teeth whitening techniques may be more natural, but results will be slow to show. If you are diligent in your use, though, and patient in waiting, you will find that these methods are the healthiest and best way to whiten your teeth.

Back in the dental care aisle, you will notice that there are a number of varying types of tooth whitening toothpastes. This is a good place to start your search for natural teeth whitening. The toothpastes, as opposed to whitening treatments, generally do use natural whiteners. They are rarely chemically based, but it is best to check out the ingredients label first to make sure. Usually the label will even let you know what the "active" ingredients are. That should make it a little easier for you to tell what the whiteners in it are. If you are unsure about what you are looking for or looking at, then do more research. In most cases, you will see bamboo powder, calcium carbonate, or silica as the whitener in your toothpaste. If it is not one of those, it is probably not natural.

As you check ingredients, there are things you should look for and others that you should look to avoid. A rule of thumb is to avoid all abrasives.

Abrasives are often used to remove stains from the teeth, but they may also remove enamel. Enamel is the outside coating on your teeth and what makes them durable, so it is counterproductive to whiten your teeth with something that damages the enamel. What you should be looking for is silica. Silica is a cleaner and whitener of teeth that removes stains. It is able to remove stains without damaging enamel because it is not a harsh abrasive.

In addition to seeking out these natural teeth whiteners, there is something else you can do. You can drink a lot of water. Not only does drinking water keep your body hydrated, but it also steers you clear of other drinks that can stain your teeth.

Coffee, tea, and dark colas are notorious for darkening teeth. Having one occasionally will not result in long-term staining, but drinking them often can cause a lot of staining problems in your mouth. Another thing you can do is stop smoking. Cigarette and Cigar smoking are not only bad for you, but they also stain teeth severely over time. Whitening teeth is not just about promotion whiteness, but also about preventing excess staining in the first place.

Maybe it's vanity or maybe it's just a desire to have healthier teeth, but either way, teeth whitening has become big business.

There are mouth washes, treatments, creams, gels, tapes, toothpastes, and even gums that claim to increase the whiteness of your teeth and remove stains. How do you sort it all out, though? If you want to avoid harsh chemicals and abrasives, it is best to make your way to the natural tooth whiteners.

Usually found in toothpaste, you should consult the active ingredient list to locate the right one for you to use. In addition, you should be looking to prevention of future discoloration and staining by drinking plenty of water and avoiding those habits that can stain your teeth.

About the Author

Sharon Douglas has a way of revolutionizing the way women look and the way they feel about beauty. Sharon is tagged as legendary in the fashion and beauty industry. Her sole mission in the beauty and fashion industry is to help women look like themselves, but better.

Sharon lives in New Jersey with her equally beautiful sister.